INTRODUCTORY ADDRESS

AT THE

OPENING OF THE THIRD SESSION

OF THE

Detroit Homœopathic Medical College,

DELIVERED BY

J. H. P. FROST, A. M., M. D.,

On Wednesday Evening, October 15th, 1873.

DETROIT:
DAILY POST BOOK AND JOB PRINTING ESTABLISHMENT.

1873.

INTRODUCTORY ADDRESS

AT THE

OPENING OF THE THIRD SESSION

OF THE

Detroit Homœopathic Medical College,

DELIVERED BY

J. H. P. FROST, A. M., M. D.,

On Wednesday Evening, October 15th, 1873.

DETROIT:
DAILY POST BOOK AND JOB PRINTING ESTABLISHMENT.

1873.

THE PHYSICIAN OF THE FUTURE.

IN the present, the future and the past, as in three great forms of life, all human interests are included. The anticipated future and the remembered past alike centre in the present, which becomes for us, therefore, *the everlasting now.* While the memories that make up the history of the past and the prophecies of the future, which express the philosophy of that history, are equally capable of aiding us in the present. That everliving present, to which each succeeding day, and every successive hour, adds its special burden of responsibilities and duties. Responsibilities and duties which, if fairly met and faithfully performed, cannot fail to bring their own exceeding great reward in the *mens conscia recti*—the personal consciousness of integrity, which shall strengthen the weary spirit; sustain the soul amid the sorrows and sufferings of this earthly existence, and keep alive within the heart the ennobling sense of constant preparation for another life and a future state more august and grand and glorious than this. For, if

"They also serve who only stand and wait,"

how much more shall not those be promoted and rewarded who devote themselves and sacrifice their lives even for the well-being and safety of their fellow men!

Many of these are found in the humbler spheres of society—heroes of conflagration and collision by land, and of shipwreck and disaster at sea; noble-hearted men, who, with their own bodies, stop the very jaws of death that others may escape. Nor should we fail to make mention here of the physicians who, in countless instances, disdaining to flee in seasons of public peril, have fought "the pestilence that walketh in darkness, and the destruction that wasteth at noon day," till, worn out with unceasing labor, day and night, they too have fallen and passed into the silent land, unnoticed and unknown! These, and such as these—brave sons of heroes—victims of unrequited toil and unselfish devotion to humanity, may indeed be forgotten in the present world; but not in that of the great hereafter. For of the least of these it is written:

> "Eternal tablets shall record
> Their names with those, who, since the world began,
> With an immortal strength, and toil and word
> Have wrought for man."

What theme, then, can be more suitable to the present occasion, or more acceptable to this audience, than that of the physician? And how shall we best discuss this great theme? Not surely with reference to the present, where praise of some, however well merited, could not but appear to disparage others equally deserving; where criticism would be invidious, and comparisons odious.

We might, indeed, call up before you the great physicians of the ages past, some of whom were priests, others princes, Archiaters, physicians to emperors, companions of kings or learned philosophers, such as Aesculapius, Hippocrates, Erasistratus, Aristotle,* Galen, Aretæus, Celsus, Oribasius and Cæsarius. Or we might invoke some of those who, in later times, became famous for the great advances they wrought in the various departments of science, and for the immense benefits they conferred upon mankind. Physicians like Van Helmont and Vesalius; Glisson and Gilbert; Haller and Hufeland and Hunter; Cullen and Cooper and Brown; Harvey and Jenner; Boerhaave and Bichat and Broussais; Rush and McClellan; Livingstone and Mott and Kane, and multitudes of others, the briefest review of any one of whose useful lives might profitably employ the passing hour.

Or, instead, we might summon before you one greater than any of these—*Hahnemann*—the illustrious founder of Homœopathy, who, within our own recollection, was gathered to his fathers; who spent long years of his early life, and no small portion of his maturer age, amid poverty and persecution and

* According to Athænaus, Aristotle, while quite a young man, kept an apothecary shop in the city of Athens.

exile, in self-denying and unappreciated labors for his fellow men. And we might picture to you the great success of his later years, and the crowning glory of his ripe old age, when, his new science of healing being at last triumphantly vindicated and acknowledged, his house in the great capitol of Europe was thronged with patients of the highest rank, both noble and royal, who sought, and in their own persons received, the proofs of his almost miraculous skill.

But to some other occasion, and to some more eloquent speaker, it must be reserved to give you the history of this sublime old man—the greatest human benefactor of humanity. For the present, therefore, we dismiss him with this brief mention. But let us not forget that in his case, as well as in that of others, "the memory of the just is blessed;" that his good deeds live after him,* and that the halo of glory that surrounds his name among men grows brighter and brighter with the advancing ages, and as he himself becomes more loved and more revered by the constantly increasing numbers of his disciples.

Just now we need to turn our thoughts in another direction. The circumstances of the past are changed. No one of the great examples we have cited is perfectly suited to present conditions, or exactly adapted to our immediate object; although many of them are eminently calculated to excite the ambition of the student and inspire his soul with high resolve. *The future alone remains.* Let me portray for you, then, *the Physician of the Future;* an ideal picture indeed, and necessarily *imperfect;* but one that may be made sufficiently *complete* for illustration, and in which, as in a mirror, may be displayed the reciprocal relations of the physician to society, and of society to the physician, and which may at the same time afford a better opportunity for presenting such considerations as may seem proper on this occasion.

But permit me to remark at the outset, that for what may be advanced in the course of this Address no one but myself can be held responsible. Should I have the misfortune to assert any-

* Denn wisse, was du auch gethan,
Du thust es auf Zeitlebens in Erinnerung;
Die gute That, klingt helle den Himmel an,
Wie eine Glocke, ja er wird zum Spiegel,
In dem du aufschauend selig dich erblickst.

thing that may be repugnant to the views of my hearers, or contrary to the truth, no blame can attach to the regular faculty of this medical college, who, while honoring me with an invitation to address you this evening, have left me entirely at liberty both as to my theme and as to the subject matter of my discourse.

I. THE PHYSICIAN OF THE FUTURE WLLL BE A MAN OF SCIENCE. Each one of the collateral branches of medical knowledge will receive his profound attention. In the *anatomy* and *physiology* of the human system, both separately and in comparison with those of the lower animals, he will be as familiar as the school boy with the rule of three. Nor will he allow himself to remain ignorant of HISTOLOGY, that new and beautiful science which explains the origin, growth and development of the different tissues composing the human body. And to this he will pay the more attention, since an accurate acquaintance with the minutest and most interior parts, of the primordial cells even, may lead to a more exact adaptation of the remedies to the disordered tissues and to the organs they compose.

Every division of *Natural Science*, the physician of the future will cultivate with the utmost zeal. Especially will he seek to learn all that can be known of those wonderful forces of nature—light, heat, gravity, electricity, magnetism, and others still more mysterious, by means of which the mechanism of the earth is maintained, and the growth of plants and the external life of animals and men supported. Nor will he be content with merely learning what is already understood of subjects like these, which are as interesting as they are important. In this, as in other directions, he will seek to extend the boundary of science, thus emulating the example of many of his predecessors who have so largely increased the amount of useful knowledge. The wondrous relations of the forces of nature to those of human life will, therefore, challenge his most serious study. Here are questions that so far have baffled the researches of scientists alike of the present and the past. And while the physician of the future may not any more than those who have preceded him arrive at the ultimate truth in this respect, he will doubtless remove much of the obscurity that has hitherto enshrouded the union of physical and vital forces; enable men to distinguish more clearly between the known and the unknown, and determine with more exactness the dividing line between the knowable and the unknowable.

In *chemistry* and in *botany*, the physican of the future will, of course, become expert. But he will be far from satisfying himself with simply ascertaining the external and physical properties and relations to each other of the various organic and inorganic substances of nature. With patient industry and life-long application he will investigate all the relations of these substances to the human system, in health and in sickness.

It is ever thus—that one science leads to others still higher. And here we see how *Pathogenesis* arises—founded on chemistry and botany on the one hand, and connected with anatomy, physiology and psychology on the other. This new science, which investigates the influences exerted on the human system by the mineral, vegetable and animal substances, was inaugurated by *Hahnemann*, and by him carried to such a degree of perfection that his followers have done little more than imitate his example; or if apparently improving upon his method, they have never surpassed him in actual results. Eminently practical in its nature, pathogenesis becomes at the same time the foundation of Homœopathy, and the basis of all that is reliable and truly scientific in therapeutics. And it is even now being cultivated with great assiduity by the most learned and enterprising of the Old School. They have, indeed, a different name, "The Physiological Method,"* but the meaning is the same. And the fact that our brethren, the most enlightened of the allopaths, as if ashamed of silently stealing our system and appropriating our medicines, are at last building up similar pathogentic foundations for themselves, should increase our faith in *Homœopathy*, and strengthen our efforts to keep the lead in this grand reformation in the theory and practice of medicine.

But little, indeed, will genuine homœopaths care how much their allopathic co-laborers convey the *thunder* of our practice, if they will but acknowledge the *lightning* of our principles. And we may state here that it is orthodox now in the Old School, to admit that the homœopathic doctrine, the law of similars, is

* Hahnemannian Monthly, July, 1873, p. 577. Dr. T. F. Allen.

indeed a real law of cure, but not the only and universal law. And the results of the great change, *from reviling to imitation*, that has come over the spirit of the Old School dream of exclusive possession of the healing art, already begin to become apparent. Statistics show that in some sections, in Philadelphia, for instance, the allopathic treatment of scarlatina is now nearly if not quite as successful as our own. And this immense improvement is simply due to the fact that, in the treatment of this disease the allopathists have followed our methods and employed our remedies, *Belladonna* in particular, which at the present time, as in that of Hahnemann, is as specific in the smooth or Sydenham variety of scarlet fever, as quinine ever is in ague.

Solomon, the wisest of the ancients, discoursed of trees, "from the cedar tree that is in Lebanon, even to the hyssop that springeth out of the wall."* So shall the physician of the future, conscious that in all the substances of nature some good and useful qualities reside, never cease his labors in the study of pathogenesis, until he has determined the virtues of all the solids, liquids and gases, and of all the vegetable and animal substances with which the earth is filled, and proved for each its exact sphere of usefulness for man. In this way remedies are obtained for all known disorders, and material provided in advance with which every new form of disease may be promptly checked at its first appearing.

In those branches of scientific knowledge which belong more nearly to the practice of medicine, *the physician of the future* can hardly fail to improve upon the present and the past. In *diagnosis* and the examination of the sick, he will be sure to employ all the recently discovered means and methods of exploration. The model husband, who now, somewhat facetiously, tells the doctor his wife is ailing and desires him to go down and *look the property over*, will then be more likely to ask him *to look it through and through!* For to the speculum and spectroscope, the ophthalmoscope, endoscope, laryngoscope and microscope, the sphygmograph and dynamograph,† the spirometer, dynamometer, galvanometer, thermometer, and various other

* I Kings, IV. 33

† Quarterly Journal of Psychological Medicine, Vol. II, p. 139.

"scopes" and "meters" too numerous to mention, of the present day, there will doubtless be added an automatic and self-recording *omniscope* and *omnimeter* combined in one, by means of which every organ and tissue in the human body may be inspected and portrayed, and every movement of muscles, every vibration of nerves, every pulsation of arteries, and every evolution of infinitesimal cell-germs even, may be duly observed, and its dynamics determined and recorded.

But even then the scientific physician, although so thoroughly armed and equipped for the detection of physical and objective symptoms, will need to study also those that are sensational and subjective. He will still need to listen to the patient's own account of the feelings and sufferings which have given rise to, or resulted from, the morbid phenomena directly perceived by his senses, or discovered by the aid of his instrumental apparatus. Consciousness and intelligence on the part of the patient will still be required, in order to show the connection of the internal and external symptoms with each other; and the physician's own judgment and experience will equally be needed to enable him to discern the true value and comparative importance of each class of symptoms in every case.

But it is not too much to affirm that the coming age may go far beyond the present, may by far surpass even the methods just described, in discovering the hidden springs of disease. Who shall say that the physician of the future may not as freely employ the wonderful faculty of *clairvoyance* to ascertain the interior constitution and condition of the sick, as those of the present day do the spirometer to measure the quantity of the air respired? Why should not this mysterious power be fully investigated and regularly cultivated in those in whom it naturally appears? Why should it not be redeemed from the suspicion of unhallowed superstition, rescued from the degrading hands of mountebanks and charlatans, and devoted to the noble uses of science and benevolence? It is not to be assumed that this remarkable faculty—which is natural to a few, and which may be acquired by many others—is ever given except for wise reasons; or that it was intended by Divine Providence to be prostituted to evil, rather than sanctified by being employed for good purposes!

With such a faculty at his command the physician of the future would have no need of our supposed *omniscope;* the patient himself, or another for him, could be made to look within, and describe with accuracy the condition and operation of the most interior organization, in connection with the accompanying sensations. Such a method, reserved perhaps for the most difficult cases, could not fail to throw great and much needed light upon those obscure forms of disease in which a morbid state of the mind results from disorders, otherwise imperceptible, of the voluntary or involuntary nervous system. In cases of this kind, and in those in which a previously existing bodily affection disappears, to be succeeded by mental or moral aberrations, nothing short of a *clairvoyant* inspection could point out the pathological condition of the delicate and subtle "membranes," "*plastic medium,*" or so-called "spiritual body," which forms the ultimate means of union between the immaterial soul and the material frame of man.

But it must not be forgotten that even at the present day, these and other forms of physical disorder, whose causes may be unknown and whose relations to physical disease it may be impossible to discover, are successfully treated by administering the corresponding homœopathic remedies—remedies whose adaptation to these mental and moral disorders is ascertained, pathogenetically, by observing their effects when taken by persons in health.

And this same clairvoyant faculty might also be applied to the investigation of the qualities and virtues of the various substances which may be employed as medicines. Such a method, if it could be reduced to practice—and why should not the future realize all that the present can anticipate?—could hardly fail to reveal, in their fullest extent, those ultimate pathogenetic powers and corresponding curative virtues of drugs, which alone are homœopathic to the most advanced forms of disease, and which are now only speculatively inferred from analogy, or imperfectly gleaned from experience. In this way the physician of the future may be enabled to see at a glance the various and most recondite medicinal qualities of substances hitherto unknown. By this cultivation of the higher powers of the soul, those of the next age may be enabled to discern by a sort of *intuitive perception* all that is now only partially learned by the slow process of induction and painful experiment. And this will be but the commencement of the return to that *instinctive knowledge* of the essential nature and relations of things, which was the birth-right of our first parents, and which enabled them to bestow upon each and every object in nature a name expressive of its true spiritual quality. But at the present day the few and scattered traces of this knowledge, which occasionally make their appearance, are scoffed at as evidences of superstition, or denounced as the fruits of sorcery.

In *pathology* the physician of the future will be well skilled. Not, indeed, in that kind so fashionable at the present day—with our allopathic brethren, especially—which occupies itself with minute descriptions of the appearance of the various tissues *after death*, which fills learned volumes with the details of the *consequences of death;* but which is as impotent to reveal the *cause* of death, as it is to save life. The true and useful pathology of the future will consist in a profound knowledge of the different morbid conditions of the whole system while living; whether these morbid conditions are confined to one tissue or organ, or embrace an entire series of organs; whether they are located in the physical, mental or moral sphere; or are equally diffused through the whole economy of the individual being.

The pathology of the future will also embrace a complete knowledge of disorders of the mind as resulting from corresponding bodily states; and will at the same time unfold, in all their varieties, the physical consequences of morbid affections of a purely mental or moral nature. And as an indispensable preliminary, this pathology, in connection with the physiology and psychology of the future, will decide the hitherto open question of the relation of the voluntary or involuntary nervous system to the various forms of disease. By means of the method of self introspection, if in no other way, the physician of the future will be enabled to determine just what symptoms belong to the voluntary, or cerebro-spinal nervous system; what to the involuntary, or ganglionic, nervous system, and what morbid phenomena indicate that both are involved together.

With such perfect pathological knowledge, the essential character of diseases, in their several manifestations, cannot but be more thoroughly understood. While the location and principal symptoms, both external and internal, of each disorder, with their producing causes, as well proximate as remote, will at once suggest the appropriate treatment and indicate the remedy which must exactly correspond to the whole case. Thus will the average duration of disease be shortened, and that of human life prolonged.

In paying the most marked attention to *hygiene,* both public and private, the physicians of the coming age will but imitate the great fathers of medicine of the remotest antiquity. Pythagoras, who lived in the golden era of the world, when medicine was not yet separated from philosophy, taught his disciples to pay supreme regard to the regulation of the diet.* And no services rendered to society by physicians or other scientific men, can equal in value those which point out the dangers that from time to time may threaten the public health. Could the physicians of Shreveport, La., have notified their fellow citizens that the method there pursued of disposing of the town sewage was dangerous in the extreme, they might have prevented the pestilence which has rendered that place the Golgotha of the South.† And just such inestimable blessings we think will be conferred upon mankind by the physician of the future, by warning communities against influences and practices which may prove destructive to the public health.

In all the departments of practical knowledge the physicians of the past, and we may say of the present also, have always signalized themselves as leaders. To them are due a great part

Medicinæ eam maxime speciem amplectebantur, quæ dietam moderatur.—JAMBLICUS, *De Vitæ Pythagoræ,* No. 163.

† A remarkable illustration of this occurred in the early history of one of the oldest homœopathic practitioners of Pennsylvania—Dr. H. Detwiller—who, by the discovery of *lead poisoning,* from apple butter kept in glazed earthen crocks, as the cause of a wide-spread epidemic, delivered thousands from a disorder which had hitherto proved incurable. As a homœopathic physician, familiar with the pathogenetic or drug action of lead, he had no difficulty in at once recognizing the nature, and ascertaining the source, of the most painful and destructive disorder that prevailed where he first settled.

of the noblest advances, and many of the most important discoveries, in those natural sciences which become the foundation of useful arts. Under the influence of dominant minds, each succeeding age has its own favorite study and field of research; each has also had its own peculiar fashion of doctrine and tone of thought. The previous age was largely devoted to natural philosophy, and many of its leading spirits openly denied, or tacitly ignored as *unscientific*, all that was not physical and material. In the present age this tendency is still manifest, although far less obtrusively so than before. Some from whom better things might have been expected, have not scrupled to claim everything for the sphere of the sensual; to repudiate all that is called spiritual or supernatural. While others even venture to assert, in so many words, *that the brain secretes thought as the liver secretes bile!**

But this doctrine is now avowedly rejected by many naturalists of the highest eminence; men like Agassiz, whose profound studies in nature have not blinded their eyes to the God of nature. Still it is not to be denied that too generally there has been shown a disposition to reckon nothing within the sphere of science that could not be measured, weighed and counted, or that does not come within the cognizance of our external senses. But the limits of human knowledge and discovery in this latter direction are already well nigh reached. And the most important problems of science, unexplained hitherto, and reserved, in part at least, for the physician of the future, relate rather to the spiritual than to the physical nature of man. They are problems that pertain, as already stated, to the *union of matter and spirit;* problems, therefore, which defy all physical calculus, whether mathematical, chemical or electrical, and which demand

* This oft quoted expression originated with *Cabanis*—born in 1757—a disciple of Condillac, and friend and relation (by marriage) of Condorcet. Similar is the doctrine of Mr. Toland (John), quoted by Haslam in his "Observations on Madness and Melancholy," London, 1809.

Cogitatio (hic minime præterunda) est motus peculiaris cerebri, quod hujus facultatis est proprium organum: Vel potius cerebri pars quædam, in medulla spinali et nervis cum suis meningibus continuata, tenet animi principatum, motumque perficit tam cogitationis quam sensationis; quæ secundum cerebri diversam in omnium animalium structuram, mire variantur.—*Pantheisticon*, p. 12.

for their solution the application of a *higher law*, that of the spiritual principle itself, which is so intimately associated with our material frame. The sphere, therefore, in which the physician of the future will achieve his greatest triumph is neither exclusively physical, nor yet purely spiritual, but, like man himself, it is a compound of the two, and its doctrine is called psychology.

This science of *psychology* is the outgrowth and ultimate development of physiology; it is the science which considers the soul of man in its connection with the body; which investigates the nature and mode of union of the human body with the human soul, and in which is studied the reciprocal influence of the body upon the spirit and of the spirit upon the body. With this wonderful and mysterious union of matter and spirit in man is connected the greater part of the hitherto undeciphered questions in philosophy; such as the doctrine of life, its identity with the soul;* the mode in which the spirit operates upon and through the body; the nature and principles of the soul's action as mechanical or otherwise, and the possibility of the spirit's ever being in this life, as the Apostle expresses it, "either in the body or out of the body."† These are the great problems of psychology, and these are the questions whose solution will in no small degree depend upon the physicians of the future; since they will at the same time interest him as a man of science, and associate themselves with him in his practical duties, and professional lite.‡

The key to many of the difficulties of normal physiology is found revealed in the phenomena of abnormal physiology, or pathology. This is plainly seen in the electro-magnetic examination of nerves, whose failure of action in disease discovers their special functions in health. In like manner the solution of many important questions in psychology—notably those relating to the union of body and spirit—can only be reached by studying the phenomena of morbid psychology, where the curtain seems partially withdrawn, and the inmost veil of the sacred temple of

* Porter's "Human Intellect," p. 36.

† I Corinthians, 15:44, and II Corinthians, 12:2.

‡ "Why should we leave an unknown quantity to the future, which, perhaps, will not consider it unknown?"—"Outlines of the Infinite," p. 100.

nature temporarily rent in twain. And it is in this direction alone that, we shall find a truly scientific answer to the materialistic tendencies and teachings of much of the so-called science of the present day.*

In the astonishing facts of natural *somnambulism*, and in those of *animal magnetism* or artifical somnambulism; in the wonderful phenomena of *clairvoyance*, including both far-seeing and prevision or "second sight," and in the still more recondite experience of those who become subject to *ecstacy* or *trance*, are seen innumerable testimonies to the power of the soul when acting in partial independence of the body. And these exhibitions of the apparent separation of the soul from the body throw more light upon the natural relation of the body to the spirit, and of the spirit to the body, than could ever be obtained from the whole science of normal psychology. These irregular and infrequent exhibitions of *spirit-power* are well calculated to strike terror into the observer's heart—powers of this kind being commonly, but incorrectly, attributed to *demoniacal* influence. Such, for example, was that wonderful display of spirit-force made by an Indian *Medicine Man*, Black Snake, of whom it is authentically related that, in a contest with a rival medicine man, concentrating all his powers, or as the Indians term it, *gathering his medicine*, he commanded his opponent to die, when the unfortunate conjuror succumbed as to a superior moral force, and his spirit, in the words of the Indian informant, *went beyond the Sand Buttes!*† Of another, it is related by a highly educated and deeply religious Catholic priest, European by birth, and formerly professor in a Continental University of high repute, that he had himself seen a Kootenai Indian command a mountain sheep to fall dead, and the animal, then leaping among the

* This materialism even in Christian lands and modern times is put to shame beside the profound philosophy and almost spiritual insight of the most ancient pagan philosophers. *Nam* MENS, ex Pythagoræ sententiæ, *cuncta cernit, cunctaque audit; Surda cœca, cetera Sunt.* PORPHYRIUS, *De Vita Pythag.* N. 47 (*Græce et Latine*) Amstelodami, 1707. "For, according to Pythagoras, THE MIND SEES ALL THINGS, AND HEARS ALL THINGS; everything else is deaf and blind."

† Atlantic Monthly, July 1866, p. 114.

Vide also "Night Side of Nature," by *C. Crowe*, Vol. 1, p. 273.

rocks of the mountain side, fell instantly lifeless. This the priest states that he saw with his own eyes, that he ate of the animal afterwards, and that it was unwounded, healthy, and perfectly wild.* These well authenticated instances I mention, out of multitudes equally astounding that might be adduced, in order to remind you that there are indeed

> "More things betwixt the heavens and the earth
> Than were dreamed of in our philosophy."

Many volumes have been published filled with narratives of this kind,—narratives attested by an ample amount of unimpeachable evidence. A great abundance of facts has been accumulated of the different classes of phenomena, just mentioned; but facts alone do not make a science, or explain their own source and origin. Some master mind is needed to perform for these mysterious operations of the spiritual world of man, the same office that *Newton* performed for the terrestrial and celestial worlds, in discovering the great law of gravitation, which applied to them all, and explained all their complicated motions,—even those in which they deviated from their exact courses. This great work, we believe, will be achieved by some physician of the future, who, laying aside on the one hand, all the grossness and unbelief of the positivists, and on the other hand avoiding alike the fine drawn speculations and abstract theories of metaphysicians, and the overweening credulity of pure spiritualists, will study these recondite mysteries of the human soul, as displayed in its irregular manifestations, with an impartial spirit, an unprejudiced mind and an all-comprehending genius, that cannot fail to lead him to success. That will demonstrate the natural law that controls the soul of man, even in its wildest vagaries; the law that binds it in its normal condition to the voluntary nervous system; that in its abnormal state—as in the case of spontaneous or induced somnambulism—transfers it for a season to the organic nervous-system, and the law, finally, that permits its apparent temporary migration from the body—as in the state of trance—and, closing the physical senses to open those which are spiritual, allows the soul to mingle and commune awhile with the inhabitants of the spiritual world itself.

* Atlantic Monthly, July 1866, p. 115.

The physician of the future, realising that body and soul are indeed *really united* in the natural state of man, and that in this profound and hitherto inscrutable union exists the key to the old-time problem of the commerce of matter and spirit, will patiently study the phenomena of this union of body and soul, as partially revealed in the counter-phenomena of their apparent separation in life. Thus will he arrive at a truly scientific and satisfactory view of their actual separation in death. And thus, too, will the physician of the future elucidate, in this and in other directions, the *fundamental principles* which shall dissipate from science the gathering clouds of materialism, and sustain rather than oppose the just claims of Religion and Revelation.* While at the same time these principles will show how such remarkable phenomena as those we have just related, *springing from causes purely natural*, have no relation to the miracles of the Sacred Scriptures. And these principles, finally, will prove that the truth of God is one and inseparable and entirely harmonious in all the various and apparently conflicting, but really corresponding spheres of physical and spiritual nature. Thus will the physician of the future, while developing the advanced science of psychology, remove from the profession the old reproach of irreligion and infidelity; contribute to reconcile reason and revelation, and establish in the last and highest achievements of science, a rational foundation for the highest faith.

But it must not be forgotten that there is another department of psychology, in which the physician of the future will preeminently show himself a man of science and skill. And this is the wide region of *morbid psychology*, the *pathology of the mind*, or disorders of the mental and moral sphere. In the physicians of the past and present, Homœopathy has indeed triumphed over the difficulties of the *bodily world* of man; has shown herself capable of vanquishing all the "ills that human *flesh* is heir to."

* "The light of the understanding is not a dry or pure light, but drenched in the will and the affections, and the intellect forms the sciences accordingly; for what men desire should be true, they are most inclined to believe. The understanding, therefore, rejects things difficult, as being impatient of enquiry; things just and solid, because they limit hope, *and the deeper mysteries of nature (it rejects) through superstition.*"—*Bacon* "Novum Organum."

But there is yet another and nobler world in man,—of mind and spirit; a world of higher human being, and profounder human suffering; a world subjected to innumerable perversions in each of its three great divisions of the *intellect*, the *sensibilities*, and the *will*. A world of *morbid perceptive*, *emotional* and *voluntary* life, in many instances disordered, depraved, almost destroyed —into which the physician of the future is summoned to enter, with silent feet, clean hands and a pure heart. Here guided by the highest intelligence, and stimulated by the most benevolent spirit, he will find ample employment for all his wisdom and all his energy.

In this great sphere of the disordered soul of man, will be found work eminently worthy the physician of the future, clothed with all the scientific advantages in which our prophetic faith and hopes have portrayed him. Hahnemann himself laid broad and deep the foundations for the greatest success here, in the minute and conscientious record of the emotional, mental, moral and volitional symptoms of the various drugs which he so laboriously proved. Some of the most convincing evidences of the truth of the Homœopathic law were found in the removal of morbid mental and moral states, by such remedies as Arsenicum, Aurum, Helleborus, Ignatia and Veratrum. And one of his own most splendid cures, one that went far to establish the new science and art of Homœopathy in Europe, was that of the famous German scholar Klockenbring, who had been deranged and confined in a lunatic asylum, and who was restored to perfect sanity.

When it is demanded of the physician of the future:

> " Can'st thou minister to a mind diseased,
> " Pluck from the memory a rooted sorrow,
> " Raze out the written troubles of the brain,
> " And with some sweet, oblivious antidote,
> " Cleanse the stuffed bosom of that perilous stuff
> " Which weighs upon the heart ?

He will answer: All this I can, and more. For he knows that far back of the actual outbreak of insanity lies the *insane temperament*, waiting but for time and favorable influences to develop itself into *Mania* or *Dementia*. He knows that in the native constitution of many, in the profoundest recesses of their organic nervous system, are deeply implanted the hereditary seeds of the various mental and moral diseases, that reduce men beneath the level of the brute. And we are well assured that the anticipation and detection of these morbid germs before they are developed, will engross all the subtle and scientific means of exploration which we have assigned him, and that their eradication will employ all the remedial agencies at his command, guided by his utmost skill. And we are equally certain that in conferring such supreme benefits upon mankind, the physician of the future will be amply rewarded for all his sacrifices, nobly compensated for all his enthusiasm and devotion; for such a consciousness of doing good, more precious than silver and gold, shall be to him *like the price of wisdom, far above rubies.**

The physician of the future must be, *facile princeps*, a man of corporeal vigor; of mental faculties strong and unimpaired, and of moral qualities at once high and elevating. Under the sure guidance of Homœopathy, by means of the dynamic virtues of her medicines, and aided by the ennobling influences of his own exalted and benevolent nature, he will be instrumental in raising the most afflicted of his fellow men, and in replacing them in that state "but little lower than the angels," in which they were originally created. Thus the physician, so often accused of materialism, indifference and unbelief, instead of the antagonist, becomes the co-laborer with those who, in circles purely religious, devote themselves to the moral and spiritual advancement of mankind. The priest, the minister and the missionary address themselves to the mind and soul; work from above downwards, and strive to purify the outward life by first renewing the indwelling spirit. The physician, on the contrary, works from below upwards; addresses himself primarily to the body, and seeks, by improving the physical and psychical condition from an external point of view, to break the shackles of *involuntary disease*, both mental and moral, and so finally to accomplish all that his sphere allows in the elevation of man as an individual and as a race.

* Job 28:18.

In this wide field of *involuntary disorder* of the mental and moral nature—based as it so largely is upon physical disease—the physician must first enter and perform his appropriate part. And when, through the united operation of all the hygienic means, medicines and moral influences at his command, he *cures* these unfortunates, so that they may be found sitting and clothed and in their right minds;* when he has thus so far elevated and transformed their degraded and depraved natures as to restore them to *voluntary and responsible* life, then he will have but prepared them for the physician of the soul, whose blessed office it is to lead them in the green pastures and beside the still waters of higher and heavenly life.

II. The physician of the future will be a man of heart. Ever conscious of the sufferings and sorrows of those to whom he is called to minister, he will deeply sympathize with them in all their misfortunes. But his sympathy will not be of the soft-hearted kind of some whom I have known, whose tears are but too ready to flow, and whose excess of feeling and tell tale countenance augment rather than assuage their patients' anxiety and distress. But it will be that silent, practical, efficient sympathy, that manifests itself in employing the best means of relief. How much true philosophy is expressed in those well known words of the old Roman:

Haud ignari malis, disco succurrere miseros.

Not unconscious of suffering, I learn to succor the miserable. And no one surely can attain to the high order of the true physician who is not tolerant of the weaknesses and follies even of the afflicted, knowing that these are often but the consequences of the physical and psychical disorders which it is at once his duty and his greatest glory to remove. Let no one, therefore, aspire to the noble office of the physician of the future who cannot, in the largeness of his own heart, appreciate to their full extent the physical and spiritual sufferings of his fellowmen; who cannot at once personally and practically sympathize with them in their distresses. This kindly, helpful sympathy forms the very life and outflowing spirit of the true physician. By

* Mark V : 15.

means of this he imparts to the sick, the feeble and the exhausted, the desponding and despairing, a strength of body and activity of mind before unknown. It is by this congenial sympathy and generous inspiration of personal vitality, that the physician of the future will most resemble that divine-human physician of souls, who when on earth did not disdain to heal the sick; who was *himself afflicted in all the afflictions of his people, and who saved them by the angel of his presence.**

In another respect, also, the physician of the future will show himself a *man of heart*, a large-hearted man. Conscious of the dignity of his calling, and profoundly impressed with the glorious destiny of his race, he will rise above all the petty strifes and contentions, the envious rivalries and low-born jealousies, which have so much discredited the profession heretofore, and from which so many of its brightest ornaments have not been exempt. Instead of hindering or opposing others in their progressive enterprises, and of imitating the example of his predecessors, who reviled and persecuted *Harvey* for discovering the circulation of the blood, *Jenner* for introducing vaccination, *Mesmer* for making splendid cures with animal magnetism, and *Hahnemann* for placing the practice of medicine on a basis truly scientific and healing the sick with infinitesimal doses; the physician of the future will welcome every one whose labors and discoveries, like those just mentioned, shall manifestly tend to ameliorate the condition of the human race And he will especially feel it both his duty and his privilege to aid in every good work for the improvement of his chosen profession, and for the better education of its future members. As a man of heart then, the physician of the future will co-operate with his fellow citizens in all their plans of charity and labors of love; sympathize with them in all the joys and sorrows that belong to the sacred ties of domestic life; partake with them in all their dearest hopes for the present world, and share with them in all their loftiest aspirations for the world to come. For thus, and thus only, can the physician of the future render himself such a minister of health as the coming age will most surely demand.

* Isaiah, LXIII, 9.

III. THE PHYSICIAN OF THE FUTURE WILL BE A MAN OF FAITH: faith in his accepted system of medical practice; faith in the medicines he employs, and faith in himself as being able to accomplish for the sick all that their case requires—all that circumstances render possible. This personal faith, founded on a substantial basis of scientific knowledge, will animate him with a confidence of success that cannot but go far to render that success assured—since it will at the same time inspire his patients with an unswerving confidence in his ability and skill. Thus will they be brought into a true magnetic *rapport* with each other, and such an intimate bond of union and spiritual sympathy be set up between them as shall render the patient a thousand times more amenable to the healing power of the physician. But in another, and still higher sense, the physcian of the future will be a man of faith. It has been the fashion with some professed men of science to ridicule religion as beneath their notice; and many others, less learned, have thought to display their consciousness of superior wisdom by dwelling upon what they are pleased to call the absurdities of Christian doctrine. Such antagonists may well expose the human errors that, in the lapse of ages, have fastened themselves upon Christianity, as barnacles become attached to the sides of a noble ship; but they can no more affect the present power, or prevent the future growth and glorious development of the purest and most truly Divine system of religion the world has ever known, than the astrologists of old could move the stars in heaven from their appointed places. Among such revilers of the highest truth, the physician of the future will not be numbered.

While not himself necessarily a sectarian, he will regard with profound respect all the different religious doctrines in which good men devoutly believe; and see, with reverence, something inspiring and truly symbolic in their various forms of worship. Thus will he naturally, it may be unconsciously, come to belong to that great *church of the future*, foreshadowed even now, which shall sustain a living *Christianity above creeds*; which shall include all the children of God, and whose members shall embody the highest faith in the humblest works of beneficence. And for the rest—without claiming to comprehend the infinite by the finite; without assuming to solve the awful problem of the origin of evil, and without even attempting to penetrate the mysteries of our holy religion, the physician of the future will be equally thankful to learn all that may be revealed of the nal verities, and content to believe where he cannot know. Conscious that as in philosophy, or natural science, there are many things not understood; so in theology, or spiritual science, there must be much that is past finding out. Thus waiving on the one hand the literalism of merely textual commentators, and on the other hand discarding the unwarranted liberties and unfounded conclusions of rationalistic expounders, he will find in the written Word a perennial fountain of Divine Truth, and dwell in that serene height of faith which shall enable him to look down upon the wickedness of mankind as a means of discipline and to be overruled for good; and to realize, despite the too apparent preponderance of falsehood and depravity, of ignorance and irreligion, that God is still in Christ reconciling the world unto Himself.

The physician who is worthy of his profession, is at the same time deeply conscious of the exalted and charitable nature of his calling. The poor, therefore, whom "we have always with us," will command his services equally with the rich; and his constant aim will be to ameliorate the condition of his fellow men, rather than to enrich himself at their expense. The daily life of the physician of the future will in this manner be filled with works of practical piety and benevolence, and inspired by an ever-increasing faith. And while thus maintaining a conscience void of offense toward God and man, he will feel that he has a right to ask for the blessing of heaven upon his efforts to heal the sick, and he will expect to see that blessing bestowed in an abundant measure. And through all the discouragements and trials that never fail to attend such unselfish labors, he will be comforted by the sense of duty performed, upheld by an unseen hand in his season of greatest need, and in his darkest hours encouraged by an unfading hope that, being found faithful in the few things of this present life, he may, at its close, be made ruler over many things in that which is to come.

Such a physician may every medical student strive to become; and such a physician may every community recognize and receive as a public benefactor.

www.ingramcontent.com/pod-product-compliance
Lightning Source LLC
LaVergne TN
LVHW011141110826
845150LV00008B/2447
* 9 7 8 1 4 1 8 1 9 3 5 3 9 *